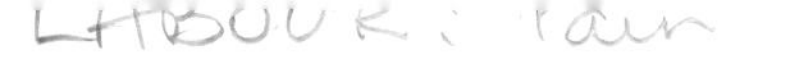

Complementary methods of controlling labour pain

Rosemary Mander

PhD, MSc, RGN, SCM, MTD

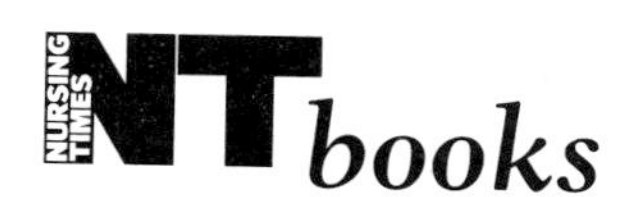

Emap Healthcare Ltd
Greater London House
Hampstead Road
London NW1 7EJ

2000

Nursing Times Clinical Monographs are authoritative, concise, single subject publications designed to provide a critical review of material that will be of value to practising nurses, midwives and health visitors. Their authors, all experts in their field, are asked to be challenging and thought-provoking and to stimulate reflection on current practice. *Nursing Times* Clinical Monographs do not seek to be exhaustive reviews but up-to-date overviews; their critical and evaluative nature is designed to promote best practice through consideration of current evidence.

Topics for publication are decided by the editorial advisory board, with input from practitioners. Monographs are then commissioned as near as possible to the publication date to ensure that the information they contain is the latest available. All manuscripts are reviewed by a board member and a clinician working in the field covered.

At regular intervals, 12–15 new monographs will be published. They will cover subjects suggested by practitioners (see below) and any major new developments in the field of nursing care. Each publication will be on sale for a limited time, after which it will be withdrawn and, if necessary, replaced with an updated version.

Note: For referencing purposes NT Clinical Monographs should be treated as books

Suggestions for future titles are welcome and should be sent to Simon Seljeflot at NT Books, Emap Healthcare, Greater London House, London NW1 7EJ

Study Hours

All NT Clinical Monographs have been given a Study Hours rating. This is an approximate guide to the amount of time it might take a nurse, midwife or health visitor with no specialist education on the subject to read and reflect on the article and consider the suggested key reading list. By doing this you can accrue Study Hours to help towards your PREP study acitivities. Make a note of any related study you undertake and keep a record in your personal professional profile. For your free Study Hours pack, call 01483 455040.

Complementary methods of controlling labour pain

Rosemary Mander, PhD, MSc, RGN, SCM, MTD

This monograph focuses particularly on pain during childbirth, although the information is likely to be relevant to painful experiences at other times during pregnancy. It also considers how ways of responding to labour pain vary according to history, culture and geography, as well as health care systems. Complementary therapies have aroused considerable interest in childbearing women and those who care for them. The meaning of the term will be examined; next, research into complementary pain control and issues associated with undertaking such research. These methods are investigated as well as the extent to which research helps both the woman deciding on her method of pain control and the midwife seeking to provide research-based information. The monograph concludes by drawing together issues a woman should bear in mind when contemplating the use of complementary methods.

Terminology

Complementary therapies are not easy to define and such definitions as do exist tend to focus on these therapies' negative attributes, such as what they are not and the personnel who do not use them (Micozzi, 1996). A more positive definition emphasises the holistic approach to health embodied by complementary therapies (Moore and Holden, 1997). These methods aim to treat the whole person, including body, mind and spirit. The complementary approaches contrast sharply with the Cartesian view of the body as a machine in which any malfunctioning part may need to be treated, removed or replaced and on which modern Western medical practice is based.

In order to further clarify the meaning of 'complementary' I build on Moore and Holden's definition by incorporating the concept of an explicit theoretical basis which differs from that generally accepted in Western health care. This theoretical basis or 'systems theory' approach (Lewith, 1998) requires that the patient, client or, in the present context, woman learns of an approach to health which is distinct from the orthodox. This process of learning may either be taught by an authority who may also be a practitioner or it may be self-taught, perhaps by reading. Invariably, though, there is a third party, who may be influential by their physical presence with the woman or through what they have taught her, either in person or through their writings.

The term 'complementary' is used here in preference to the frequently used 'alternative'. The latter term is a 1960s throwback, relating to 'drop-outs' and their life-styles. Further, 'alternative' suggests an exclusive divide between conventional Western medicine and complementary therapies. To emphasise the existence of this divide is unhelpful and may be inaccurate. The term 'alternative' is particularly inappropriate in the present context because of the complexity of labour pain, derived as it is from a number of sources. It has been observed that in certain pain experi-

Notes

ences it is not possible for one therapy on its own to achieve resolution (Chapman, 1990). For this reason Melzack and Wall believe it is fully justified to use a combination of therapies (1991). Labour is likely to be one of these situations, and the use of one approach to control the pain does not exclude the possibility of others being used simultaneously. Thus, these approaches are more accurately described as complementary rather than alternative.

The evidence base

For the woman considering using any method of pain control in labour there are a number of features about which she will need information in order to make her decision. Obviously one of these is the effectiveness of the intervention. Another, less frequently mentioned, is the 'disutility' of the intervention (Vickers, 1999) by which is meant its harmfulness, invasiveness or inconvenience. Expense may also need to be included as a disutility. Thus, these are areas about which the woman and her carers may require research-based information.

The questions that arise in relation to research on these issues are whether such research is feasible and, if so, whether it constitutes evidence. In this area the difficulties of undertaking randomised controlled trials (RCTs), widely regarded as the gold standard in terms of evidence, are manifold (Vickers, 1999). It is necessary to ask, though, whether this standard is an absolute requirement in the context of pain control in labour. Part of the answer to this question may be found in the more general context of care in labour, where examples of inadequately researched yet widely used interventions abound (Mander, 1999). Additionally, although the RCT may be an ideal tool for the assessment of the effectiveness of an intervention such as pain control, it may be less appropriate to assess the more woman-oriented aspects of that intervention which Vickers has referred to as 'disutility'. The question of the need for evidence is further answered by the limited availability of evidence to inform clinical decision-making. It has been estimated that only about 12% of our clinical or management decisions are able to be informed by sound evidence (Page, 1996). Even with the passage of time since this estimate, I would suggest that a majority of decisions still lack an evidence base.

It is not possible to conclude that the lack of research into these methods is due to lack of interest. A more likely explanation emerges in the work of North American authors such as Micozzi (1996) and Spencer (1999). Inevitably drawing on their experience within the US health care system, these authors indicate the insurance companies' unpreparedness to meet the costs of complementary pain control. The absence of obstetrics and childbearing from these research-based texts on complementary health care shows that this observation applies as much, or more, in maternity care than in other areas of health care. Even though the insurers' decision may have been taken on the basis of the lack of research evidence to support the use of these methods, it has the effect of limiting the use of and, hence, further research into complementary methods. This is an example of what has become known as 'insurance-led health care' (Mander, 1997). Thus, the development of knowledge is effectively stifled in a country which is a major contributor to the health care knowledge base, and this inevitably has an impact on other developed countries' maternity care provision.

One question that arises from contemplating the need for evidence relates to the nature of the research which constitutes the evidence base. Although I have referred to RCTs as the gold standard, it is not impossible that other, possibly less 'scientific', forms of research are well able to provide the answers the woman and her carers need to enable her to make sound decisions relating to her requirement for pain control (Lewith, 1998; Dimond, 1998).

The uncertain relevance of the RCT in this context derives not only from its narrow focus on specific outcomes.

Notes

As mentioned already, complementary therapies comprise a holistic orientation which address the individual's unique situation. This applies as much to the pain of labour as it does to any other health condition. For this reason, as Vickers emphasises, the inputs into the therapy vary according to the client's individual characteristics, such as her personality or her taste in food (Vickers, 1999). The inputs are also likely to vary according to the individual practitioner's theoretical background. For example, some acupuncturists rely heavily on the traditional Chinese medicine (TCM) concepts of yin and yang; others, on the other hand, have incorporated aspects of Western neurophysiology into their practice (Vickers, 1999).

Complementary methods

In considering complementary methods it is necessary to be selective, as the list runs into hundreds of different therapies (Dimond, 1998) and may even be infinite. This is partly because of the dynamic nature of the phenomenon, as innovative methods are publicised and gain interest, adherents and significance. This changing picture may present a challenge to the practitioner attending the woman in labour. It is likely, however, to benefit the woman seeking a method of pain control suited to her personal childbearing experience (Mander, 1998). Thus, the list here does not claim to be exhaustive but includes those methods most commonly used (Royal College of Midwives, 1999).

In order to examine the multiplicity of complementary methods of pain control available to the woman in labour, it is helpful to use a theoretical framework. The one used here is based on the positive effects of the woman assuming some control over her childbirth experience (Mander, 1992; Green et al, 1990). Thus I seek to address the following aspects of each method:

- The control of pain or its effectiveness;
- The control over the progress of labour, that is, whether any delay or dystocia is likely to ensue;
- The effect on the developing relationship between the mother and baby through fetal and/or neonatal effects;
- The woman's control of her own behaviour, that is, her self control.

The mode of action is discussed only briefly, as this tends to be less than certain in the context of the complementary therapies and depends to a large extent on the theoretical basis underpinning the intervention. Information relating to the mode of action of pain control interventions is available elsewhere (McCrea, 1998; Mander, 1998).

Acupuncture

The origins of modern acupuncture may be traced back to classical TCM with its underlying principle of health comprising a balance between the opposing energy forces (Bensoussan, 1991). Acupuncture needles are inserted at recognised points along designated meridians of the body, with the aim of allowing noxious air to escape from the affected body part. In this way, cleansing is sought and balance should be restored. The acupoint BL-32 (*ciliaou*), which overlies the second sacral foramina, is believed to control the pain of childbirth, especially back pain (Deadman et al, 1998).

The availability of this form of pain control in the UK emerged in a large-scale nation-wide study of pain control in labour (Steer, 1993). This showed that out of the 291 maternity units that responded to the survey questionnaires, nine (3.3%) offered women acupuncture either alone or in combination with relaxation and/or hypnosis.

An accurate assessment of the effectiveness of acupuncture in dealing with pain in labour may be prevented by the lack of properly designed and implemented RCTs (Porter, 1997). An example is found in a planned two-stage study of acupuncture in labour involving, first, volunteers and, second, randomisation (Wallis et al, 1974). The poor results of stage one, in

Notes

which 90% of women found the analgesia inadequate and 76% required other forms of analgesia, meant that stage two could not go ahead. In spite of these poor outcomes, approximately one-third of the women were sufficiently positive about acupuncture to state that they would choose to use it again in a future pregnancy.

These positive impressions, in spite of less than consistent, predictable or adequate analgesia, were also found in the study by Abouleish and Depp (1975). Of the 12 women in the study, nine considered the analgesia provided to be adequate and would be happy to use it again. The reasons for these positive reactions related to the lack of sedation or other side-effects and to the lack of medication which might affect the fetus. While the effectiveness of acupuncture may be uncertain, the lack of any diminution of the mother's self-control is regarded as desirable. The researchers identified that the acupuncture interfered with electronic fetal monitoring, but whether this interference had any implications for the fetus is not clear.

The effects of acupuncture on the progress of labour have more recently become apparent in the work of Zeisler and colleagues (1998). These researchers' retrospective study showed that the acupuncture group of women (n=57) experienced a median duration of labour of 196 minutes compared with 321 minutes for the non-acupuncture group (n=63). Unsurprisingly, in the non-acupuncture group the women were significantly more likely to have their labour augmented with oxytocin.

The use of acupuncture by UK midwives is recounted by Robotham (1998) with an emphasis on the benefits during pregnancy rather than on the control of labour pain.

Aromatherapy

The application of highly concentrated essential oils by massage, inhalation, dropping on to the skin or other routes has been proposed as a means of alleviating a range of conditions, including pain. The mode of action is uncertain, but the production of endorphins by stimulation of the olfactory nerve is one possibility (Porter, 1997). Another is the activation of the 'old' part of the brain, the limbic system, to achieve more psychotropic effects (Moore and Holden, 1997).

Research into the benefits of aromatherapy is not plentiful, but an example is found in the study by Wilkinson (1995) which featured the administration of 1% Roman camomile by massage. Both the control group and the experiment group showed a reduction in anxiety, although there was a greater reduction in the group whose massage involved an active essential oil. The extent to which the researcher was able to 'blind' the masseuse is not clear, but this aspect may reduce the value of the findings.

In Oxford, Burns and Blamey undertook a pilot study of the use of aromatherapy in labour involving 585 selected women (1994). There was no control group. The essential oils used included peppermint, eucalyptus, frankincense, clary sage, jasmine, camomile, rose, lemon, mandarin and lavender. Although some essential oils, such as lavender, camomile and jasmine, have been claimed to have analgesic effects (Moore and Holden, 1997), Burns and Blamey do not claim such properties. A range of effects were identified for the various preparations, including acceleration of labour, relaxation and analgesia. The most frequent indication for the use of aromatherapy was reduction of anxiety, followed by treatment of nausea, stimulation of uterine contractions and pain control in that order.

A spontaneous vaginal birth was achieved by 71% of the women. The results show that the essential oils were perceived by both mothers and midwives as most effective in assisting relaxation, treating nausea and vomiting and enhancing the woman's mood. While lavender and clary sage were often regarded as helpful in accelerating labour, the perceptions of effects varied between women and between women and midwives. Analgesic effects varied similarly.

Burns and Blamey's study gives an overall picture of the women and midwives being satisfied with the use of aromatherapy, to the extent that the service was continued after completion of the study owing to demand. A majority of the women (62%) considered that the use of essential oils was effective, whereas for only 12% of women were they regarded as ineffective. These authors do not mention any fetal effects. The Caesarean rate (8%) and the instrumental birth rate (20%), however, suggest that such effects, if any, were minimal. Effects on the woman's self-control are not mentioned either. That the woman was more likely (than the midwife) to mention that her mood had been 'enhanced' may indicate that such enhancement was not unwelcome.

Homoeopathy

In the 19th century Samuel Hahnemann made the observation that 'like cures like' (Hahnemann, 1983). He was referring particularly to a substance that causes a particular symptom in healthy people being used to cure a disease characterised by that symptom (Castro, 1992). Steer (1993) found that homoeopathy was used for pain control by 22 women in a sample of 6,093 (0.4%). Homoeopathy is thought to have its effect by stimulating the body to correct a problem itself, such as by bringing the immune system into action to cure an infectious condition.

One homoeopath (Smith, 1998) discusses the benefits of using arnica during labour to control the woman's pain, based on her experience as a homoeopath. This use of arnica is followed by continued administration for three days postnatally to ease discomfort and promote healing. Smith warns against the prophylactic use of caullophyllum to make labour easier, owing to the possibility of sensitivity to this powerful preparation.

An example of homoeopathy which has attracted much attention is the Bach flower remedies (Trevelyan, 1994). These are intended to help the user to cope with a range of difficult emotional states. Their attraction may possibly be due to these remedies' ease of self-diagnosis and self-prescription.

Research has yet to establish the efficacy of homoeopathic remedies for labour pain (Porter, 1997; Smith, 1998). This verdict is supported by a systematic review by Kleijnen and colleagues (1991), who examined the evidence for the efficacy of homoeopathy using controlled trials. In total, 107 controlled trials were found to have been published world-wide. The researchers were scathing in their assessment, stating that 'most trials seemed to be of very low quality, but there were many exceptions' (Kleijnen et al, 1991). While warning the reader of the likelihood of publication bias, these researchers identified a beneficial trend regardless of the quality of the trial or the form of homoeopathy used. Of the 105 trials with interpretable results, 81 indicated beneficial effects, whereas in 24 no benefits of homoeopathy were found. These researchers conclude that there is a strong case for further evaluation of the therapy but only by well-conducted trials.

It is usual to assume that small quantities of greatly diluted, relatively benign substances are unlikely to affect the fetus, the progress of labour or the woman's self-control. It is necessary, however, to recall Smith's (1998) warning against the prophylactic use of caullophyllum on the grounds of its power and thus its potential for harm. It may be that this assumption of harmlessness in homoeopathy, as in other complementary therapies, may not always be appropriate (Spencer, 1999).

Hypnotherapy

Hypnosis is probably best known for its ability 'to induce states of selective attentional focusing' (Taylor, 1999). The benefits of hypnotherapy in labour, however, are thought to rely on its facilitation of relaxation .

Although research on hypnotherapy

Notes

in labour has been undertaken, it demonstrates a number of weaknesses. The randomised controlled trial by Freeman and colleagues (1986) used epidural administration as the proxy measurement for the experience of pain. This less than satisfactory proxy measure enabled these researchers to conclude that there was no difference between the group that had been taught self-hypnosis and the control group. Freeman and colleagues made no attempt to assess the susceptibility of the women to hypnosis or 'hypnotisability' (Spanos et al, 1994), which may partly account for the lack of inter-group difference. That only 15% of the population, and presumably the sample, are easily 'hypnotisable' may be the reason for these inconclusive results.

This problem was addressed by a study of the effects of hypnotherapy in combination with childbirth education (Harmon et al, 1990). The volunteer sample comprised 60 primigravid women. The women's hypnotic susceptibility was assessed and they were grouped accordingly (high/low susceptibility) before receiving six childbirth education sessions. These groups were further randomly subdivided, so that half of the women in each group were taught hypnotic induction at the beginning of each session. The researchers found that the women who had been taught self-hypnosis reported less pain, experienced shorter first stages, used less analgesic medication, gave birth to babies with higher Apgar scores and were more likely to give birth spontaneously than those in the control groups.

Harmon and colleagues' finding of the effect of hypnotherapy on the duration of labour has been endorsed by a larger and more local study (Jenkins and Pritchard, 1993). The sample comprised volunteers of whom 126 were primigravid women with 300 age-matched controls and 136 were women having their second baby with 300 age-matched controls. Recruitment was by inviting women attending antenatal clinics to undergo hypnotherapy. The mean length of the first stage of labour in the primigravid women was significantly shorter in the hypnotised group (6.4 hours compared with 9.3 hours in the control group). The mean length of the second stage was also significantly shorter in the experiment group (37 minutes compared with 50 minutes). In the parous women the corresponding values were 5.3 hours and 6.2 hours and 24 and 22 minutes. The use of analgesic medication was significantly reduced in both hypnotised groups compared with their controls. The value of this study, however, is reduced by the researchers including only those women who gave birth spontaneously in the data analysis.

Hypnotherapy is another example of the literature concentrating little attention on the fetal effects of the pain control intervention. The effect on the woman's self-control, though, may be uncertain, especially in view of the bad press that hypnosis tends to attract.

Acupressure (shiatsu massage)

Many complementary therapies, including acupressure, therapeutic touch, massage and reflexology, require the use of the therapist's hands. That feature may be the only one they share, as the knowledge base underpinning each therapy is likely to derive from very different origins.

The theoretical framework described for acupuncture also applies to the practice of acupressure. The difference lies in the approach to the points on the meridians which, rather than needles being inserted, have digital pressure applied or are massaged. Although there are a few accounts of the relevance of acupressure in labour (Moore and Holden, 1997; Yates, 1998), it is hard to identify any relevant research reports. Moore and Holden suggest that acupressure may be more appropriate in controlling labour pain because, unlike acupuncture, the presence of a therapist is not required. Clearly the woman who chooses to use acupressure in labour needs to learn this therapy, probably being taught by an acupuncturist before the onset of labour.

Notes

An example of research into the use of acupressure which may be relevant to the present context was undertaken by Ho and colleagues (1996). These researchers investigated the effects of stimulation of the P-6 (*neiguan*) acupoint. This point, situated on the inner aspect of the wrist, is one of the traditional Chinese acupuncture points and is widely used for anti-emetic purposes (Deadman et al, 1998). The study focused on women given epidural morphine for post-Caesarean pain control. A double-blind RCT involved 60 women, who were allocated to have the acupressure bands or placebo bands applied on the P-6 acupoint bilaterally before the Caesarean. The incidence of nausea and vomiting was significantly decreased. Vomiting occurred in 27% of the controls but in none of the acupressure group. The randomisation of the women should have overcome any cultural bias owing to this study having been undertaken in the Republic of China.

Therapeutic touch

The theoretical basis of therapeutic touch (TT) originated in the orient and seeks to transfer 'life energy' (*prana* or *chi*) from the healthy practitioner to the patient or client to resolve a health problem (Meehan, 1998). Whether TT merits discussion here is debatable. The first reason is that it may not be a 'manual' therapy owing to the absence of physical contact between the practitioner and client, giving rise to the name 'non-contact therapeutic touch' (O'Mathuna, 1999). Second, the ability of TT practitioners to detect 'life energy' has been questioned (Rosa et al, 1998), as have the claims of benefits (Claman, 1994).

In contrast to these criticisms, the almost evangelical claims made by Krieger (1997) for the efficacy of TT have fuelled the controversy still raging among US nurses. Although much of the research on TT has related to its effects on wound healing, some has focused on the alleviation of pain. While the pain of tension headache has been found to be significantly reduced by TT (Keller and Bzdek, 1986), postoperative pain was not affected (Meehan, 1998). In her review of non-pharmacological methods of pain control in labour, Simkin (1989) concluded that TT is an apparently harmless intervention. Thus, the effects of TT for the woman and baby have yet to be shown to be anything other than benign.

Massage

As a complementary therapy, massage now suffers from the bad press that hypnosis has long endured. In spite of this adverse publicity the study by Steer (1993) found that women stated that they had used massage as frequently as epidural analgesia (n=1178; 19.3% of mothers). Unfortunately this study did not differentiate between shiatsu, osteopathy, Swedish massage and back-rubbing or 'counter-pressure'.

Steer is critical of midwives for not including massage as a method of pain control, which accounts for the discrepancy between the midwives' reports and those of women. This omission may be due to the routine, almost unthinking use of massage in the form of 'back-rubbing' by midwives. Such uncertainty may be resolved by an inclusive definition: 'Massage is the application of hand pressure to soft tissues, usually muscles, tendons or ligaments, without causing movement or change in position of a joint in order to decrease pain, produce relaxation and/or improve circulation' (Mander, 1998).

Based on her experience of teaching couples 'Swedish' massage for labour, Smith makes certain claims for this intervention (1997). These include control of pain, relaxation, improvement in fetal oxygenation and enhancement of uterine contractions to accelerate labour. The research literature relating to massage, however, does not mention its use in childbirth. The research tends to have involved patients experiencing long-term pain, such as that resulting from cancer, on the basis of which Taylor (1999) concludes that massage is an

Notes

effective adjunct to standard care in the reduction of anxiety and self-reported pain.

In her review of the literature on 'physical methods' of pain control Porter (1997) includes osteopathy and refers to a large US study of this intervention in labour. The results were clearly beneficial to the women, as 81% experienced some relief from their pain. Additionally, the fetal benefits would have been considerable, as the women in the experiment group were administered 30% less pethidine.

Reflexology

In some ways reflexology may be comparable with acupuncture and acupressure, but it perceives the body in terms of 'zones' rather than meridians. These zones end at the feet and hands, which are the focus of the reflexologist's intervention to correct the balance of energy flow. When balance is achieved, tension, and hence pain, is thought to be reduced (Royal College of Midwives, 1999). Authoritative research into reflexology has involved patients with neurological disorders with invariably positive outcomes (Diamond et al, 1999).

A study of the effects of foot reflexology, which may be relevant in the present context, was undertaken among 130 postoperative women (Kesselring et al, 1998) who were randomised into three groups. For five days each woman received 15 minutes of foot reflexology, foot/leg massage or talking, respectively. The foot reflexology group recovered from their surgery more quickly than the other two groups, with the exception of sleep patterns which were more unsatisfactory. Of particular interest in the present context is the finding that the foot/leg massage group showed significantly better results in their subjective measurements of well-being, pain and sleep.

Music

Although not included in the Royal College of Midwives list of commonly used therapies (1999) and not mentioned by Steer (1993), it is my observation that music is a ubiquitous feature of labour wards. It may be necessary, however, to distinguish between the music that features so prominently in the labour suite and audio-analgesia. The distinction lies partly in the preparation of the woman by the therapist in order to 'render meaningful the most limited responses' (Kneafsey, 1997). Music therapy is further distinguished by the 'route of administration' which should be by headphones or an earpiece in order to exclude extraneous sounds and allow the woman control over the volume (Zimmerman et al, 1981).

Childbearing-related research is limited, but an RCT involving 54 pregnant volunteers (Sammons, 1984) produced generally favourable but not significantly different findings between music and no-music groups. In their small study (n=30) Durham and Collins (1986) identified a reduction in medication use in the sample. On the basis of a case study of a woman who used music in labour Stevens (1992) found benefits for staff as well as the mother, who particularly appreciated the increase in her personal control.

The research into music therapy in the care of people with long-term pain is of a more convincing quality and would seem to indicate effectiveness (Schorr, 1993; Beck, 1991). The findings of a study of the acute pain of postoperative obstetrical and gynaecological patients (Locsin, 1981) are both persuasive and authoritative. The music group women showed fewer overt pain reactions and used less analgesic medication than the controls.

The literature invariably refers to recorded music. Olson suggests that in childbearing experiences live music may prove to be of even greater benefit than that which has been recorded (1998).

Meditation

The patterns of breathing ordinarily taught in childbirth education may be combined with meditation to increase the woman's relaxation in labour (Moore and Holden, 1997).

Transcendental meditation relates more closely to my definition of complementary therapies in terms of a theoretical framework. Unfortunately it has not been possible to locate any relevant research on meditation.

Implications for the woman

In her attempt to help women to 'choose wisely' Thomas (1999) discusses the implications of complementary therapies for the woman involved. The benefits that Thomas lists include the woman assuming more control over her own health and the likelihood of the woman learning to 'listen' to her own body. Thomas also warns that there may be dangers of which the woman should be aware. These include the common assumption that natural equates with benign. The possibility of the manual therapies causing painful damage is also considered as a danger. Further, Thomas advises that the composition of remedies should be scrutinised, as with any product. This author also recommends the principle of 'less is more', that is, using the remedy only until the point when improvement begins.

Conclusion

This review of the research literature on complementary pain control methods supports the general impression that the research evidence is not sufficient to encourage women to rely on these methods as consistently effective. The literature which has led to this verdict, however, has also presented a picture of women's general satisfaction with these methods, despite their questionable and variable effectiveness. The limited 'disutility' of these methods compares favourably with the established harmful side-effects of many of the pharmacological methods of pain control which have been described in terms of iatrogenesis (Mander, 1998). Further, it may be that a higher standard of evidence is required of complementary therapies than of more orthodox interventions.

In support of this inequity, a member of the Research Council for Complementary Medicine has observed: 'I need more evidence that there's a unicorn in my garden than I do for a sheep' (Vickers, cited by Driscoll, 1997).

The complementary therapies discussed here are those that correspond to the definition introduced at the beginning of this monograph. For this reason a number of non-pharmacological methods have not been included. Examples are the widely used transcutaneous electrical nerve stimulation (TENS) (Carroll et al, 1997) and hydrotherapy (Lewith, 1998). Other examples would be methods which are probably even less frequently used, such as biofeedback (Duchene, 1989), Alexander technique (Diamond et al, 1999), distraction and guided imagery (Fordham Dunn, 1994). Meanwhile, an increasing number of commentators (Hughes, 1999) are recognising midwifery care as an 'intervention' that, while in no way meeting this monograph's criteria for being complementary, has been shown to reduce a woman's need for pharmacological pain control. NT

Notes

Notes

References

Abouleish, E., Depp, R. (1975) Acupuncture in obstetrics. *Anesthesia and Analgesia*; 54: 1, 82–88.

Beck, S. (1991) The therapeutic uses for cancer-related pain. *Oncology Nursing Forum*; 18:;8, 1327–1337.

Bensoussan, A. (1991) *The Vital Meridian: A Modern Exploration of Acupuncture*. Melbourne: Churchill Livingstone.

Burns, E., Blamey, C. (1994) Using aromatherapy in childbirth. *Nursing Times*; 90: 9, 54–60.

Carroll, D., Tramer, M., McQuay, H. et al (1997) Transcutaneous electrical nerve stimulation in labour pain: a systematic review. *British Journal of Obstetrics and Gynaecology*; 104: 2 ,169–175.

Castro, M. (1992) *Homeopathy for Mother and Baby*. London: Macmillan.

Chapman, C.R. (1990) Psychologic and psychosocial techniques. In: Bonica, J.J., Loeser, J.D., Chapman, C.R., Fordyce, W.E. (eds) *The Management of Pain* (2nd edn). Philadelphia, Pennsylvania: Lea and Febiger.

Claman, H.N. (1994) *Report of the Chancellor's Committee on Therapeutic Touch*. Denver, Colorado: University of Colorado Health Sciences Center.

Deadman, P., Al-Khafaji, M., Baker, K. (1998) *A Manual of Acupuncture*. Hove: Journal of Chinese Medicine Publications.

Diamond, B.J., Shifflet, S.C., Schoenberger, N.E et al (1999) Complementary/alternative therapies in the treatment of neurologic disorders. In: Spencer, J.W., Jacobs, J.J. (eds) *Complementary/Alternative Medicine: An Evidence-Based Approach*. St Louis, Missouri: C.V. Mosby.

Dimond, B. (1998) *The Legal Aspects of Complementary Therapy Practice: A Guide for Health Care Professionals*. Edinburgh: Churchill Livingstone.

Driscoll, M. (1997) Trust me, I'm a guru. *Sunday Times*; May 18, 15.

Duchene, P. (1989) Effects of biofeedback on childbirth pain. *Journal of Pain and Symptom Management*; 4: 3, 117–123.

Durham, L., Collins, M. (1986) The effect of music as a conditioning aid in prepared childbirth education. *Journal of Obstetric, Gynaecological and Neonatal Nursing*; 15: 3, 268–270.

Fordham, M., Dunn, V. (1994) *Alongside the Person in Pain*. London: Baillière Tindall.

Freeman, R.M., Macaulay, A.J., Eve, L. et al (1986) Randomised trial of self-hypnosis for analgesia in labour. *British Medical Journal* (Clinical Research Edition); 292: 6521; 657–658.

Green, J.M., Coupland, V.A., Kitzinger, J.V. (1990) Expectations, experiences and psychological outcomes of childbirth: a prospective study of 825 women. *Birth*; 17: 1, 15–24.

Hahnemann, S. (1983) *Organon of Medicine* (6th edn) (1st edn published 1810). London: Gollancz.

Harmon, T.M., Hynan, M.T., Tyre, T.E. (1990) Improved obstetric outcomes using hypnotic analgesia and skill mastery combined with childbirth education. *Journal of Consulting and Clinical Psychology*; 58: 5, 525–530.

Ho, C.M., Hseu, S.S., Tsai, S.K., Lee, T.Y. (1996) Effect of P-6 acupressure on prevention of nausea and vomiting after epidural morphine for post-cesarean section pain relief. *Acta Anaesthesiologica Scandinavica*; 40: 3, 372–375.

Hughes, D. (1999) Midwives and women coping with pain together. *Practising Midwife*; 2: 5, 12–13.

Jenkins, M.W., Pritchard, M.H. (1993) Hypnosis: practical applications and theoretical considerations in normal labour. *British Journal of Obstetrics and Gynaecology*; 100: 3, 221–226.

Keller, E., Bzdek, V.M. (1986) Effects of therapeutic touch on tension headache pain. *Nursing Research*; 35: 2, 101–106.

Kesselring, A., Spichiger, E., Muller, M. (1998) Foot reflexology: an intervention study. *Pflege*; 11: 4, 213–218.

Kleijnen, J., Knipschild, P., Ter Riet, G. (1991) Clinical trials of homoeopathy. *British Medical Journal*; 302: 6772, 316–323.

Kneafsey, R. (1997) The therapeutic use of music in a care of the elderly setting: a literature review. *Journal of Clinical Nursing*; 6: 5, 341–346.

Krieger, D. (1997) *Therapeutic Touch Inner Workbook: Ventures in Transpersonal Healing*. Santa Fe, California: Bear and Co.

Lewith, G. (1998) Misconceptions about research in complementary medicine. In: Vickers, A. (ed.) *Examining Complementary Medicine*. Cheltenham: Stanley Thornes.

Locsin, R.G.R.A.C. (1981) The effect of music on the pain of selected post-operative patients. *Journal of Advanced Nursing*; 6: 1, 19–25.

Mander, R. (1992) The control of pain in labour. *Journal of Clinical Nursing*; 1: 3, 219–223.

Mander, R. (1997) Choosing the choices in the USA: examples in the maternity area. *Journal of Advanced Nursing*; 25: 6, 1192–1197.

Mander, R. (1998) *Pain in Childbearing and Its Control*. Oxford: Blackwell Science.

Mander, R. (1999) Care in labour. In: Marsh, G., Renfrew, M.J. (eds) *Community-Based Maternity Care*. Oxford: Oxford Medical Publications.

McCrea, H. (1998) Scientific background. In: Mander, R. *Pain in Childbearing and Its Control*. Oxford: Blackwell Science.

Meehan, T.C. (1998) Therapeutic touch as a nursing intervention. *Journal of Advanced Nursing*; 28: 1, 117–125.

Melzack, R., Wall, P. (1991) *The Challenge of Pain.* Harmondsworth: Penguin.

Micozzi, M.S. (1996) *Fundamentals of Complementary and Alternative Medicine.* New York and Edinburgh: Churchill Livingstone.

Moore, S., Holden, M. (1997) Complementary medicine for pain control in labour. In: Moore, S. (ed.) *Understanding Pain and Its Relief in Labour.* Edinburgh: Churchill Livingstone.

O'Mathuna, D. (1999) *Therapeutic Touch for Wound Healing* (Cochrane Review). In: Cochrane Library: Cochrane Collaboration; Vol. 3 (Oxford Update Software).

Olson, S.I. (1998) Bedside musical care: applications in pregnancy, childbirth and neonatal care. *Journal of Obstetrical, Gynecological and Neonatal Nursing*; 27: 5, 569–575.

Page, L. (1996) The backlash against evidence-based care. *Birth*; 23: 4, 191–192.

Porter, J. (1997) Physical methods of pain relief. In: Russell, R., Scrutton, M., Porter, J. (eds) *Pain Relief in Labour.* London: British Medical Journal Publishing Group.

Robotham, M. (1998) Piercing the pain. *Nursing Times*; 94: 13, 30–32.

Rosa, L., Rosa, E., Sarner, L., Barrett, S. (1998) A close look at therapeutic touch. *Journal of the American Medical Association*; 279: 13, 1005–1010.

Royal College of Midwives (1999) Position Paper 10a: Complementary Therapies. *RCM Midwives' Journal*; 2: 12, 382–384.

Sammons, L.N. (1984) The use of music by women during childbirth. *Journal of Nurse-Midwifery*; 29: 4, 266–271.

Schorr, A. (1993) Music and pattern change in chronic pain. *Advances in Nursing Science*; 15: 4, 27–36.

Simkin, P. (1989) Non-pharmacological methods of pain relief during labour. In: Chalmers, I., Enkin, M., Keirse, M.J.N.C. (eds) *Effective Care in Pregnancy and Childbirth: Volume II.* Oxford: Oxford University Press.

Smith, J. (1998) Using homoeopathy during pregnancy and labour. *Journal of the Association of Chartered Physiotherapists in Women's Health*; 82: 1, 25–28.

Smith, R. (1997) Massage for labour. *MIDIRS Midwifery Digest*;7: 4, 434–435.

Spanos, N.P., Carmanico, S.J., Ellis, J.A. (1994) Hypnotic analgesia. In: Wall, P.D., Melzack, R. (eds) *Textbook of Pain.* Edinburgh: Churchill Livingstone.

Spencer, J.W. (1999) Essential issues in complementary/alternative medicine. In: Spencer, J.W., Jacobs, J.J. (eds) *Complementary/Alternative Medicine: An Evidence-Based Approach.* St Louis, Missouri, C.V. Mosby.

Steer, P. (1993) The availability of pain relief. In: Chamberlain, G., Wraight, A., Steer, P. (eds) *Pain and Its Relief in Childbirth: The Results of a National Survey Conducted by the National Birthday Trust.* Edinburgh: Churchill Livingstone.

Stevens, K.M. (1992) My room — not theirs! A case study of music during childbirth. *Journal of the Australian College of Midwives*; 5: 3, 27–30.

Taylor, A.G. (1999) Complementary/alternative therapies in the treatment of pain. In: Spencer, J.W., Jacobs, J.J. (eds) *Complementary/ Alternative Medicine: An Evidence-Based Approach.* St Louis, Missouri: C.V. Mosby.

Thomas, P. (1999) Choosing alternatives. *AIMS (Association for Improvement in Maternity Services) Journal*; 11: 3, 9–10.

Trevelyan, J. (1994) Homoeopathy. *Nursing Times*; 90: 4, 56–58.

Vickers, A. (1999) Editorial: evidence-based medicine and complementary medicine. *American College of Physicians Journal Club*; 130 (March–April), A13–14.

Wallis, L., Shnider, S.M., Palahniuk, R.J., Spivey, H.T. (1974) An evaluation of acupuncture in obstetrics. *Anesthesiology*; 41: 6, 596–601.

Wilkinson, S (1995) Aromatherapy and massage in palliative care. *International Journal of Palliative Nursing*; 1: 1, 21.

Yates, S. (1998) Supporting women with shiatsu — another tool for keeping birth normal. *MIDIRS Midwifery Digest*; 8: 4, 422–424.

Zeisler, H., Tempfer, C., Mayerhofer, K. et al (1998) Influence of acupuncture on duration of labor. *Gynecologic and Obstetric Investigation*; 46: 1, 22–25.

Zimmerman, M. (1981) Mechanisms of pain and pain therapy. *Triangle*; 20: 1/2, 7–18.

Literature search

The author of this monograph has attempted to ensure that the review of the literature is as comprehensive and current as possible. To this end, in addition to books and journals, the electronic databases CINAHL, MEDLINE, BIDS and PubMed as well as the MIDIRS Midwifery Digest were consulted. The search words used included 'complementary', 'alternative', 'pain' and 'labour'.

Notes

Notes

Notes

Notes